Self Healing Guide

TIBETAN SECRETS

5 STEPS TO UNLIMITED ENERGY AND RESTORED HEALTH

Mary Solomon

TABLE OF CONTENTS

Introduction

Imagine, just for a moment – visualize the Himalayas – mighty, majestic, snow clad....and a feeling of tranquility and bliss enveloping us. We all yearn to go there and experience the serenity, the peace that is a part of this beautiful place. Someday (we make a mental promise to ourselves).... someday we will take a break from our hectic schedules and spend some time amidst the beauty of the Himalayas and discover our inner selves. No family to take care of, no demands to be met, no deadlines – just one resolute soul determined to spend some time experiencing bliss, joy, silence and solitude amidst nature.

Sounds like a farfetched dream and we briskly shake our heads as reality jolts us back to earth and we go about the business of leading our lives. Is this state of mind really so elusive? Can we not experience bliss, stillness of mind and a calm and composed outlook in our daily lives? Most of us have heard about yoga and meditation. We know someone who practices it regularly and are fully aware of all the health benefits of yoga. But we feel it is too idealistic and very impractical to incorporate it into our daily schedules. Or that we need to learn it from a yoga practitioner or join a class. Exercising in the gym, too, requires time and money. So we just keep postponing the inevitable.

Until a day arrives, when we lose your temper for no concrete reason, or those aches and pains have developed into acute problems and we feel we have reached our physical, mental and emotional threshold. We decide that the least we can do is make a beginning somewhere. We weigh the pros and cons of our particular situation and want to go in for something which is not time consuming, yet gives us all the benefits of exercising. We look for ways and means of doing something which will not cost us a lot of money. And with a little research, we will realize that the Tibetan rites meet all of our requirements completely.

The Tibetan Rites has been practiced for over 2000 years. These five simple steps have proven to slow the aging process, help produce and restore energy and lead to restored health. These five simple steps can change your life.

The History Of The Five Tibetan Rites

There is an interesting story behind the Tibetan rites: 2500 years ago, a boy called Peter Kelder is believed to have lived in the mid – west United States. Some people believe that he was an adopted child and left home as a teenager. During his travels, Peter met a retired British army colonel named Colonel Bradford, in Southern California. Colonel Bradford narrated his traveling experiences to Kelder.

When the Colonel was posted in India, the natives told him about a group of lamas who seemed to have discovered the 'fountain of youth'. They told him that old, stooped men who walked with the support of a cane were transformed into healthy, strong and virile men who could walk without any support after their stay in the lamasery.

Colonel Bradford searched for the lamasery after his retirement and lived with these Tibetan monks/lamas. These Tibetan monks taught him the five Tibetan rites or exercises. They are similar to the yoga postures practiced widely in India, but the Tibetan rites emphasize movements, whereas the yoga postures are mainly static.

The Lamas explained the concept of the seven chakras or psychic vortexes to the Colonel. These chakras are actually spinning electromagnetic fields of different colors and fill us with energy as they spin. These chakras are located above the major endocrine glands of the body. Enough evidence has been found to prove that the hormones produced from these endocrine glands regulate the aging process.

These chakras should ideally be spinning in synchronization at top speed. But stress, old age, faulty diet, faulty eating habits, improper food combinations, etc. cause these chakras to spin at a slower pace.

Practicing these five simple movements boosts the spin rate of these chakras, which normalizes the hormonal imbalances of the body resulting in improved health and longevity. It makes the person feel energetic and fills him with a sense of vitality and well-being.

Practicing the five Tibetan rites daily stimulates all the seven chakras and makes them spin rapidly at the same rate. When one of these chakras is blocked, the natural spin rate slows down, thereby blocking the flow of vital life energy or prana. When the circulation of this life energy is blocked, illness, stress, aging, pain, etc. is experienced.

Colonel Bradford was also taught a sixth rite. But the Lamas recommend this rite only for those who are willing to practice celibacy.

These Tibetan rites were first publicized by Peter Kelder in 1939, in a 32 page booklet titled, "The Eye of Revelation". In this booklet, Kelder discusses his interaction with Colonel Bradford, who gives simple, precise, detailed instructions on how the Tibetan rites need to be practiced.

The emphasis on following a particular breathing pattern is not clearly implied in the original booklet. Later editions by other people recommend following a particular breathing pattern for better results and also have a word of caution for people with certain specific health conditions.

Practical Advantages Of The Five Tibetan Rites

- It requires a minimum of only 10 minutes and a maximum of twenty minutes of our time. The benefits are really worth the time.

- It doesn't cost any money.

- These movements are easy to understand and learn. We do not need an expert to guide us.

- The best part is – we can practice these movements without stepping out of our homes, but also if we are traveling.

- We can reap the benefits of the Tibetan rites by doing it indoors, regardless of the weather conditions outside.

- The Tibetan rites do not require any special equipment.

- All we need to do is spread a rug or blanket or towel on the floor.

- We need just enough space to lie down and move our arms and legs.

These Tibetan rites can be practiced at any time of the day or evening. (The benefits are enhanced if the rites are performed at day break and at sun set - but we can really do them whenever it is convenient for us).

Recommendations For Beginners

- Avoid doing these exercises on a full stomach.

- Wear loose, comfortable clothes.

- It is advisable to do them in a well ventilated area (outdoors if possible – but not in the hot sun).

- Start these exercises at a slow pace initially.

- Follow the order of the exercises.

- Initially start by performing each Tibetan rite 3 times in one day.

- Listen to your body. Avoid straining your body.

- Refrain from holding on to a position if you feel any pain or think that you may injure yourself.

- You may feel a little sore initially, but by the next day you will be fine.

- After a week's interval, increase the number of repetitions for each rite to 5.

- Keep adding 2 repetitions per week till you reach 21 repetitions per day.

- Once your body has gained strength and endurance, it will take you less than 20 minutes in all to do all the 21 repetitions for each rite.

- Improve the speed with which each exercise has to be performed gradually.

- It is more important to do the exercises correctly than to do them quickly, but incorrectly.

- Ensure that you follow the breathing pattern correctly.

- Holding your breath during the exercises or improper breathing patterns may lead to tiredness or light headedness.

- Ensure that you take at least three cleansing breaths after each exercise.

- The essence of the healing powers of the five Tibetan rites lies in holding the position for at least 2 or 3 seconds.

- Try to do these exercises at least five times in a week.

- It is better to do fewer repetitions of all the exercises every day than postponing it to another day when you have time for the entire regimen.

- Each rite should be repeated to a maximum of 21 times only.

- Avoid over doing these exercises.

- These rites are essentially for restoring the energy flow of our body, which indirectly benefits us in various ways.

- If you want to do more than 21 repetitions, adding another session later on during the day can prove to be beneficial.

- Refrain from doing these rites in the late evening or just before you go to bed.

- The 5 Tibetan rites should ideally be done after your morning shower.

- If the 5 Tibetan rites are done correctly, you should not perspire at all.

- Showering after doing the 5 Tibetan rites will prove to be ineffective as water dissipates all the prana/life energy that the exercises have built up in the body.

- It is advisable to perform these 5 Tibetan exercises in the early morning as they boost the metabolism of the body for the rest of the day and burn more body fat.

These rites will fill you up with energy that lasts for hours. While this is a great way to start the day, performing these rites in the late evening will result in building up a lot of energy for hours and we may find it difficult to fall asleep at night.

The Five Tibetan Rites of Rejuvenation

The exercises are physical demanding, but supply the body with energy for hours. The Tibetans feel that these physical movements are not exercises and prefer to call them rites. So we will use the term the five Tibetan rites throughout this book.

The First Rite/ Clock-Wise Spin

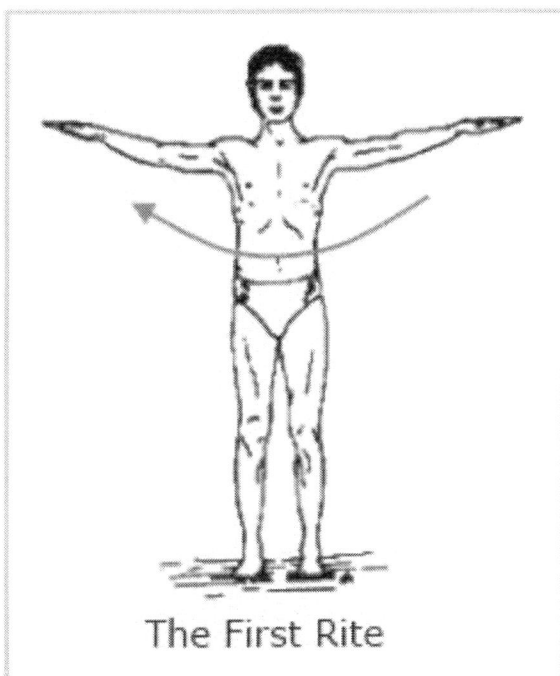

The First Rite

Stand straight keeping your spinal cord erect.

- Stretch your arms ensuring that they are straight and parallel to the floor.

- Your palms must be facing downwards with the fingers close together.

- Inhale deeply through your nose during the first spin

- Assuming that the floor had a clock on it, start spinning around very slowly in the clockwise direction until you complete 3 spins initially.

- Ensure that you are spinning around on the same spot.

- Exhale deeply through the mouth.

- After each cycle of 3 spins, place your hands on your hips with your feet apart.

- Breathe naturally.

- Begin with three spins and slowly work up to 21 repetitions.

- Look at a particular point steadily if you are feeling dizzy.

- Take two slow deep breaths after you finish this rite while you feel the sensations in your body.

- Relax for a few seconds before you start the second rite.

- Begin with three and gradually work your way up to 21 repetitions.

Benefits:

- Refreshes and revitalizes the body.

- Enhances the coordination and balance of the body.

Harmonizes the spin rates of all the chakras.

The Second Rite/ Raised Legs

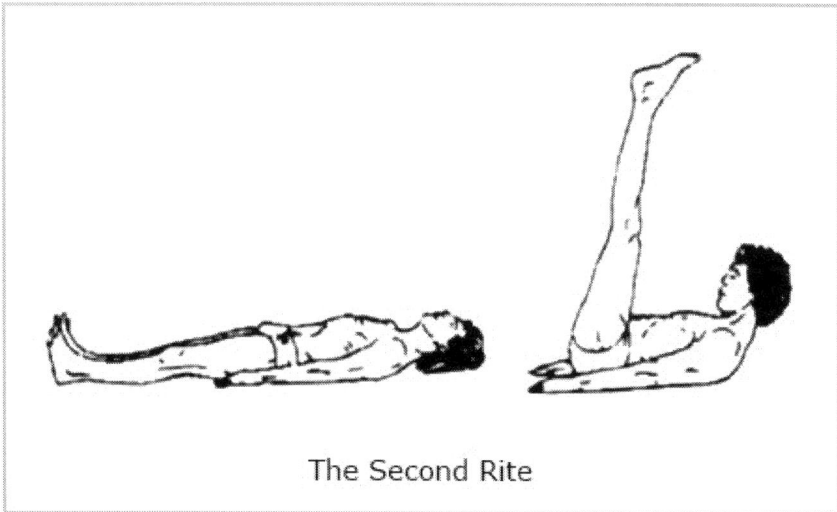

The Second Rite

- Lie down flat on the mat placed on the floor, keeping your face upwards.

- Ensure that your arms are straight and parallel to your body.

- Let the palms touch the mat and ensure that are fingers are close together.

- Take a deep breath through your nose.

- Slowly, lift your head away from the floor and bring it against your chest.

- Ensure that the chin touches the chest.

- Simultaneously, lift your legs away from the floor while keeping them straight (No bending at the knees.)

- Lift your legs till they are at 90 degrees to your body.

- Try to move the legs further (bending at the hips, not the knees) and bring them towards your head, but do not let the knees bend.

- Gradually, lower the head and the legs to the floor.

- Let the muscles relax as you exhale through the mouth.

- Inhale and exhale deeply twice after you complete each exercise.

- Take two deep breaths after you finish this rite and feel the sensations in your body.

- Relax for a few seconds before you start the third rite.

- Begin with three and gradually work your way up to 21 repetitions.

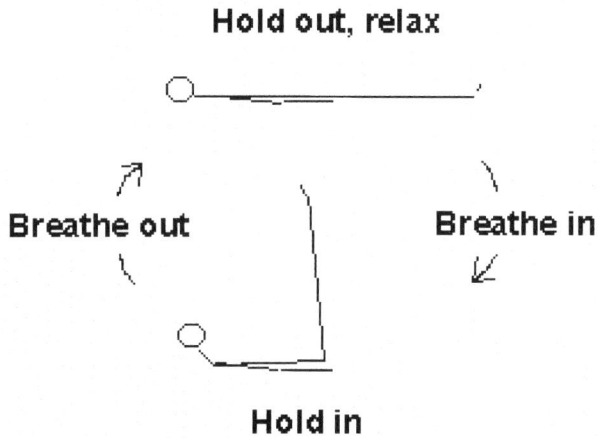

Hold out, relax

Breathe out

Breathe in

Hold in

Benefits:

- Improves clarity of mind and instills a sense of calmness and peace.

Strengthens and tones the hips, lower back, legs and neck.

The Third Rite/Back Bend On Knees

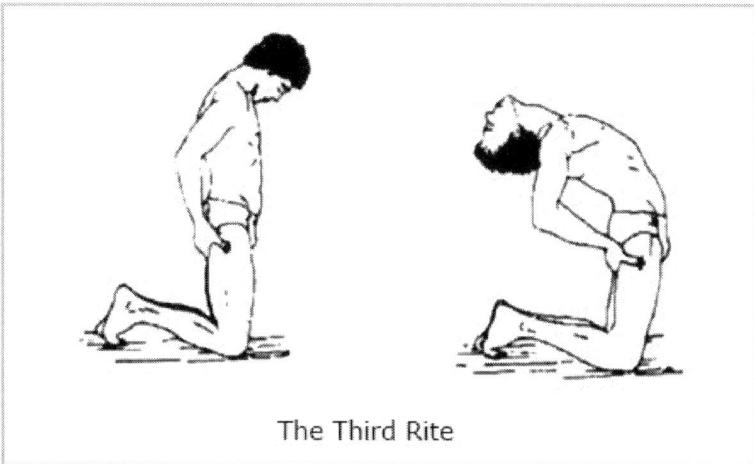

The Third Rite

- Kneel down on the mat which is placed on the floor, knees slightly apart, toes curled, keeping your spinal cord straight.

- Place your hands against your thigh muscles.

- Bring the head and neck forward to make it touch the chest.

- Ensure that the chin touches the chest.

- Take a deep breath through your nose.

- Fill your lungs completely with air.

- Take your head and neck backwards now, arching the spine.

- As your shoulder blades come together, try to bend the head and the neck backwards as far as you comfortably can.

- You can feel your lower spine relaxing.

- Support your arms and hands by placing them against the thighs as you bend backwards.

- Avoid bending beyond the waist level.

- Do not strain yourself unduly.

- Return to the original position of your chin touching your chest.

- Breathe out through the mouth.

- Your lungs should be thoroughly empty when you reach the original position.

- Take two deep cleansing breaths between each repetition.

- Take two deep breaths after you finish this rite and feel the sensations in your body.

- Relax for a few seconds before you start the fourth rite.

- As with the other rites, start with three and work your way up to 21 repetitions.

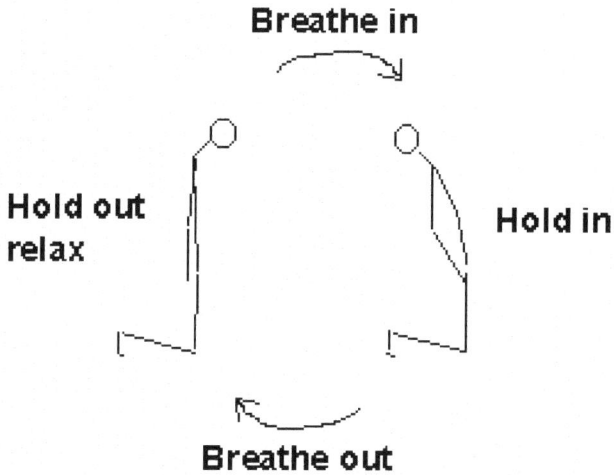

Breathe in

Hold out relax

Hold in

Breathe out

Benefits:

- Makes the body flexible.

- Enhances receptivity of mind.

- Boosts the energy flow to the heart chakra.

- Gives relief from muscle tension.

- Stretches the muscles.

Lengthens and tones the spine.

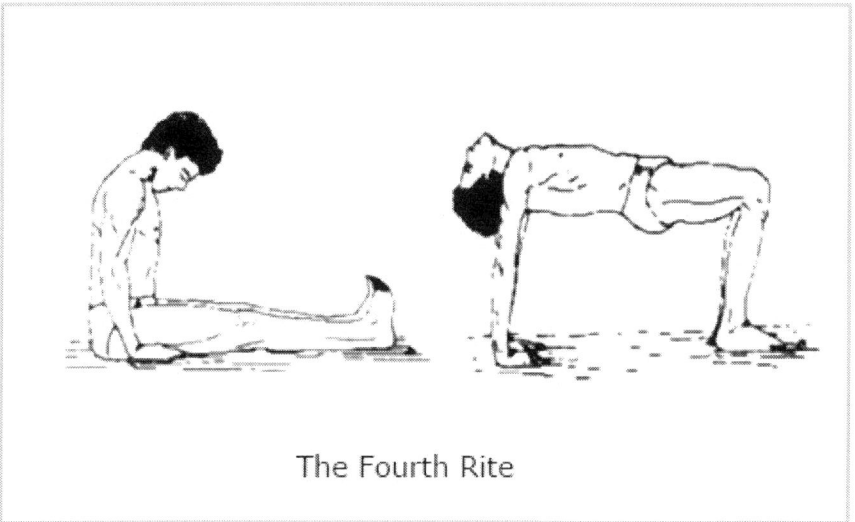

The Fourth Rite

The Fourth Rite/Table top

- Sit straight up on the mat and keep your legs outstretched in front of you.

- Ensure that your feet are around 12 inches apart.

- Let your palms rest on the mat, fingers together, near your buttocks.

- Bring your chin forward so that it rests against the chest.

- Take a deep breath through your nose.

- Now, take your head backwards fully.

- Simultaneously, raise your buttocks and bend your knees as raise your body.

- The weight of your body will automatically shift to your arms.

- Using your arms for support, continue to raise your buttocks until your midsection and thighs are straight and parallel to the floor.

- Allow your head to arch backwards as much as you possibly can.

- Now, your body will be supported with your arms and lower legs only.

- Hold your breath as you feel the tension in every muscle of the body.

- Breathe out completely through your mouth as you lower your body to the floor.

- Return to the original sitting position allowing your chin to touch your chest.

- Inhale and exhale deeply twice as you rest between repetitions.

- Take two deep breaths and feel the sensations in your body.

- Relax for a few seconds before you start the fifth rite.

- Begin with three and gradually work your way up to 21 repetitions.

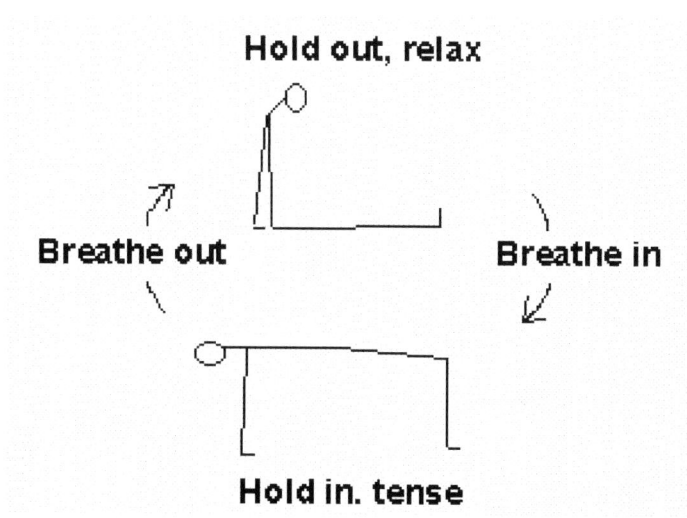

Hold out, relax

Breathe out

Breathe in

Hold in. tense

Benefits:

- Stimulates the hormonal glands.

- Enhances the stability and balance of the entire body.

- Improves the functioning of the circulatory and lymphatic systems.

Strengthens the wrists, arms, shoulders and lower body.

The Fifth Rite/ Pendulum

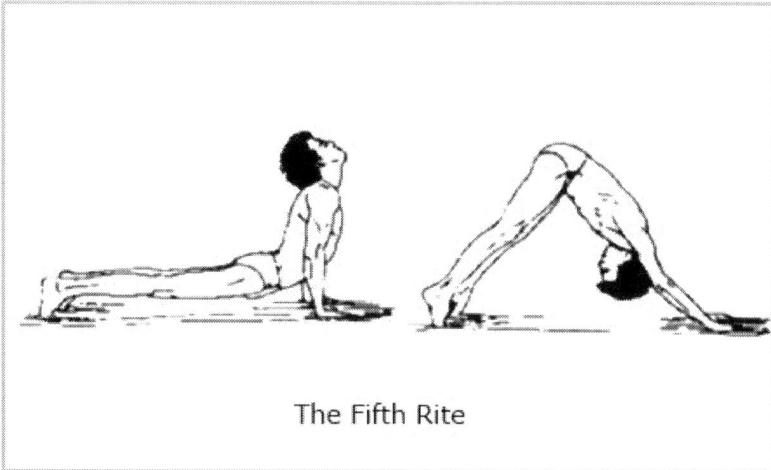

The Fifth Rite

- Position your body such that if faces downwards towards the floor.

- Ensure that your hands and feet are always straight while performing this movement.

- Breathe in deeply through your nose.

- Flexing your toes and using your arms for support, raise your body away from the floor as your arch your spine (like push- ups).

- Keep your head straight/Look directly in front of you.

- Slowly bend your head backwards.

- Except your curled toes and your arms, no part of your body should be touching the ground.

- Raise your hips gradually, push your buttocks up into the air and lift the entire body to form an inverted V shape.

- Ensure that your legs and arms are straight.

- Bring the head forward ensuring that the chin touches the chest.

- Try to make the soles of your feet touch the floor completely.

- Breathe out slowly as you lower your body.

- Return to the original position slowly (arms supporting your weight and head held backwards.

- Take two cleansing breaths between each movement.

- Begin with 3 and gradually work your way up to 21 repetitions.

- Take two deep breaths and feel the sensations in your body.

- Lie down flat on the mat on your stomach with your arms stretched out in front of you, head on one side and your eyes closed.

- Relax completely and allow your heart beats and breathing to return to normal.

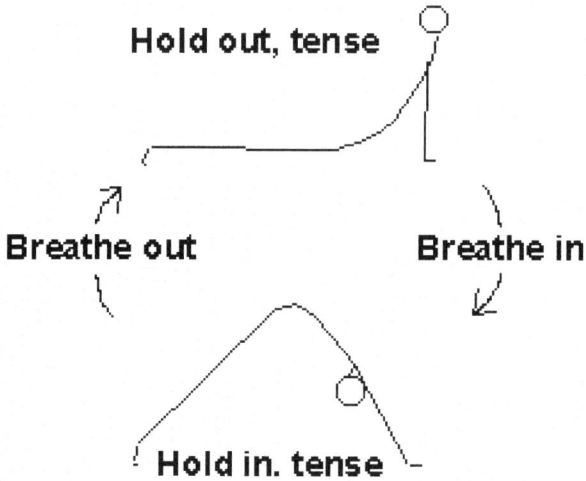

Hold out, tense

Breathe out

Breathe in

Hold in. tense

Benefits:

- Energizes the body.

- Gives us relief from fatigue and stress.

- Enhances the flexibility of the body and makes almost every muscle of our body strong.

- Motivates us to pursue this form of exercise regularly.

What to do after you finish doing the five Tibetan rites:

- The 5 Tibetan rites can be performed as a standalone form of energizing yourself or...

- You can perform these exercises as a way of warming up for any other form of exercise.

- After you finish performing these exercises, walk around for a couple of minutes or do some light stretching exercises before you go about your daily activities.

- Some people prefer to meditate after performing the Tibetan Rites. This has proved to be an excellent way of enhancing the benefits of the five Tibetan rites.

A word of caution:

- People suffering from high blood pressure and heart problems must do rite 4 and 5 very slowly and ensure that they keep their head above the level of the heart.

- People who are on drugs that cause dizziness or are suffering from health conditions like heart problems, arthritis of the spine, high blood pressure, vertigo, hyperthyroid, etc. should consult their physicians before they start doing these exercises.

Overweight people should refrain from doing rite 4 and 5 till they have developed ample physical endurance and strength.

Benefits Of The Five Tibetan Rites

When all the five exercises are repeated 21 times, the benefits are immense.

- Reduced stress: You'll feel calmer as a person and are able to deal with stressful situations coolly.

- Increased energy in the body and mind: The energy that you get from performing the five Tibetan rites lasts for hours and is unlike the caffeinated boost of energy which exhausts us after a short while.

- Enhanced feeling of calmness, mental focus and clarity of thought: We are able to retain our composure during stressful times and think clearly.

- Increased physical strength: These rites energize us thereby we don't feel exhausted or fatigued by physical work.

- Sharper memory: Reduced stress has a positive impact on our retention power leading to better memory power.

- Enhanced oxygen consumption by the body: The body consumes more oxygen when we take deep breaths while performing the rites.

- Improved respiration: With the additional oxygen that our body gets, our respiratory system is able to function more effectively.

- Weight loss around midsection: Some people find it easier to lose weight after performing the five Tibetan rites because they crave healthier foods. Other people feel this is an excellent way of controlling their weight.

- Improves muscle strength: After performing the five Tibetans, you may see your muscles building up on your arms, hips, legs, stomach and back. It tones flabby arms and tightens the abdominal muscles.

- Strengthens the spine: These movements give us relief from chronic back ache.

- Deep restful sleep: Some people experience dreamless sleep while others have more vivid dreams.

- Relief from arthritis: When the prana/life energy flows freely through the body, people suffering from arthritis get a lot of relief from their joint pains.

- Builds up the stamina, endurance and immunity of the body: We don't seem to get sick as frequently and don't fall prey to common colds as easily.

- Improves circulation of the blood.

- Improves the efficiency of the heart.

- Relaxes the nervous system: We no longer suffer from mood swings and these exercises make us feel more in control of our emotions.

- Enhanced potency/sexual performance.

- Restoration of hair.

- Anti-aging – makes you look youthful.

- Improves bone mass.

- Decreased pain.

Better digestion and elimination.

The Science Behind The Benefits

A combination of the five Tibetan rites followed by a session of meditation enhances the benefits that we gain after we do the five Tibetan rites. Scientific studies have proved that meditation is beneficial to the human body.

- In the year 2005, the Dalai Lama was invited to the annual meeting of the Society for Neuroscience in Washington D.C. During his speech, this great Tibetan spiritual leader emphasized the similarity between the Buddhist teachings and neuroscience.

- According to neuroscience, meditation is actually a series of mental exercises which gives us the necessary mental strength to control the working of our own brain. Sufficient evidence has been gathered to prove that meditation and exercise has immense direct and indirect benefits on our body.

It is now an accepted fact that there are tangible and intangible forces that are constantly working within our bodies and minds. Regular deep meditation improves the electromagnetic rhythm of the neurons and they start vibrating rapidly in harmony. That is why meditation is said to improve mood and health.

The Sixth Rite

In the booklet titled "The Eye of Revelation" that was published in 1939, Colonel Bradford reveals to his students the existence of a sixth rite that can be done if they want to gain super powerful benefits and experience mysticism.

Colonel Bradford mentions in this booklet that the benefits of these five Tibetan rites are immense, and make one appear younger and more energetic, but if a person yearns to be young in the truest sense of the world, then he should learn the sixth rite.

In order to learn the sixth rite they:

- Would have to perform 21 repetitions of the first five Tibetans properly and gain all its benefits.

- Would have to lead celibate lives.

It must be kept in mind however; that the monks who taught Colonel Bradford the 5 Tibetan rites were all male and were spiritually inclined. Celibacy was something that they had always been practicing.

Celibacy is not a choice that many men would opt for and just doing 21 repetitions of the five Tibetan rites is enough to experience the immense benefits mentioned in the booklet.

This does not necessarily mean that the sixth rite is not worth practicing. Most people are content leading normal, healthy and meaningful lives and are satisfied with the benefits of the first five Tibetan rites.

Most people who really yearn to master the technique of the sixth rite either want to at least attempt it and experience its benefits or are interested in researching the traditional Tantric practices.

In the booklet, "The Eye of Revelation" Colonel Bradford offers a word of caution for people who are keen on learning the sixth rite. He says:

"It is mandatory that a man be full of masculine virility in order to perform the sixth rite. He needs to transmute the procreative energy and for this to happen he needs be virile. It is impossible for an impotent man or a man with little virility to do the sixth rite. If he attempts to do so, it will have disastrous consequences which may end up harming him thus leading to discouragement.

If he is really keen on mastering the sixth rite, he should first practice the other five rites consistently till he experiences the power of his virility. When he experiences the first "full bloom of youth" he can go ahead and learn the sixth rite."

In the sixth rite, the sex currents of the body are upturned – i.e they are made to flow in an upward direction. The Colonel insists that the practitioner must be absolutely sure that he wishes to lead the life of a mystic. He must be absolutely sure in his mind and in his heart that this is what he desires in life, and then go ahead and learn the sixth Tibetan rite. The benefits of the sixth rite are bound to benefit him.

The essence of the sixth rite:

The colonel goes on to explain the essence of the sixth rite in detail in the booklet. He says that:

- The life energy/prana flows in the downward direction in average virile men.

- In order to gain super powers or mystic powers, these life forces need to be turned in the upward direction.

- Turning these powerful life forces in an upward direction is actually a very simple matter if done under expert guidance.

- Men over centuries have made futile attempts to master this procreative life energy force by either suppressing it or dissipating it.

- The key lies in transmuting it while simultaneously lifting it upward.

- When the sixth rite is practiced correctly, this life force is used effectively (not suppressed or dissipated) and the practitioner would have discovered the "elixir of life".

- This was something that even our learned well versed ancestors were unable to do or experience.

- The sixth rite must be performed only when the student has an excess of procreative energy which can be gained by practicing the first five Tibetans rites consistently.

- The sixth rite is very easy and can be performed at any time anywhere.

- It is imperative that the complete sequence of breathing exercises be repeated three times after doing the sixth rite.

How the sixth rite works:

- We have more than 72,000 nadis in our body. The life energy/prana flows through these nadis.

- Kundalini is a reservoir of psychic energy that is found at the base of our spine. It is coiled up like a snake.

- When the Kundalini awakens, we experience a sense of pure joy, love and knowledge.

- Our consciousness expands as we become aware of the Divine Truth.

- We have three bandhas in our body: the mula bandha, the uddiyana bandha (6th rite) and the jalandhara bandha.

- These three bandhas function as energy valves for the life energy/ prana that flows within our body.

- When these three bandhas are activated by the Tibetan exercises, during meditation or while practicing other yoga postures or breathing practices the Maha bandha is formed.

- When these bandhas work together, the blocked life energy/prana is released and it starts flowing freely nourishing that particular area.

- These bandhas also bind the life energy/prana within the body to avoid dissipation.

- This life energy/prana gets redirected within our body, thereby healing and rejuvenating us.

- When this life energy/prana starts flowing freely and in the correct direction, it makes us aware of the neuro-physical and mental energy patterns of our physical body.

- The Uddiyana bandha(sixth rite) is a valve that opens upwards during the flow of life energy.

- While doing the sixth rite, the blocked energy starts flowing upwards.

- When this energy starts flowing upwards, the psychic energy that is stored in the Kundalini is released.

- It can now flow freely and a direct connection is established between the base chakra and the chakra located in the crown.

A word of caution:

- The expert guidance of a highly competent spiritual teacher is recommended while practicing this sixth rite.

- This rite involves the nervous system and if done incorrectly or without expert supervision one may experience mental instability or psychic disturbances leading to mental stress and suffering.

The connection between tantra and the sixth rite:

There seems to be a strong connection between tantric practices and the sixth Tibetan rite. A person practicing tantra uses the life energy/prana that flows through his own body and through the universe to achieve purposeful goals. The goals differ from person to person. Some people crave for material success while others yearn for spiritual progress. Most tantric practitioners feel that it is absolutely necessary to know and learn about mystical experiences.

The tantric practitioner uses Yoga, mantra chanting, mudras (hand gestures) meditation, mind training techniques etc. to enhance the flow of prana/life energy. These practices should be made available only to students seeking advanced knowledge and who already have sound knowledge of basic practices. These advanced tantric practices should be done under the expert guidance of a guru to understand their potential.

Without the guidance of an expert, these tantric practices are likely to be misused or misinterpreted, which may prove to have disastrous consequences affecting the mental equilibrium and health of a person.

In fact, most tantric practices are kept a secret, mainly because they should never be practiced without proper guidance. Most people cannot even comprehend the symbolic and psychological impact that these practices have on one's body, mind and health. It is easy to misunderstand and misinterpret these practices and dismiss the guidance of an expert as unnecessary.

Modification Of The Five Tibetan Rites

- One must always keep in mind that the original book was published in 1939 and Colonel Bradford learned these rites from the Tibetan monks who lived in the Himalayas. The level of their physical fitness must have been extremely good in order to survive the harsh weather conditions there.

- They cultivated and cooked their own food, which was totally organic, and all their physical activity kept them in top form.

- They probably started practicing these Tibetan rites from a very young age.

- In comparison, we seem to have led a sedentary life style and are not as physically fit as our ancestors.

- So these rites have gradually been modified to suit individual needs.

- Colonel Bradford makes a mention of this in the booklet and says that a few people create their own little supports or aids to help them while practicing these movements, and it is perfectly fine to do so.

- He narrates an example of an old Indian man who just couldn't get the correct posture of the fourth rite even once. He would not be content with just lifting his body off the floor. He wanted it to parallel to the floor exactly like the rite prescribed. So he started working with a ten inch tall box which was about two and a half feet long. He padded it with bedding. He then lay down flat on his back on the bed with his feet and hands touching the floor at either end. Now he found it extremely easy to lift his body to the horizontal position. Colonel Bradford endorses modifying the exercises to suit the requirements of our body as long as the core of the exercises is not tampered with.

- As long as no radical changes are made that may have an adverse effect on the spin rate of the chakras, it is okay to modify them as per our bodily requirements.

- It is imperative that we remember one fact: The prime priority of any form of exercise, including the five Tibetan rites, should be safety and achievability.

- Several thousands of people practice the modified forms of Tibetan rites regularly.

- When broken down into a series of steps, they build up our strength gradually and safely.

- Right from day one, the prime focus should always be on correct alignment. This way, we learn to perform the exercises correctly and prevent the occurrence of muscular imbalances.

- A gradual build up of our core stability takes place. This activates the deepest muscles of the trunk while protecting and stabilizing the spine.

- The modified exercises prevent us from straining or injuring our lower back or neck.

- When we build up our strength gradually, we learn to do the movements using our strength and coordination instead of relying on the momentum of the movement.

Additional energy breathing sessions enhances the effect and impact of the five Tibetan rites on our body.

Conclusion

A visit to the Himalayas may perhaps be a distant and farfetched dream for many of us. But it is possible to incorporate some peace and some tranquility into our hectic lives. It is definitely possible to experience a slice of the Himalayas every day. We can transport ourselves mentally to the Himalayas and experience a state of bliss by following these movements. These Tibetan rites energize us and help us cope with the challenges of our daily lives with equanimity. Simply invest 10 minutes and 5 simple steps for unlimited energy and restored health. You're worth it!

If you enjoyed this ebook, please take the time to share it with your friends and post a positive review on Amazon. I would greatly appreciate it!

Crystal Healing Energy

Gemstones For Attracting Wealth and Reducing Stress

BY MARY SOLOMON

Table of Contents

An Introduction To Crystal Healing

Crystals have been used for healing purposes for over 30,000 years. Crystal healing is a non-invasive alternative treatment that works holistically to harmonize the body, mind, spirit, and emotions while helping to increase feelings of well-being, lift depression, and neutralize negativity.

How is a rock able to hold energy and heal? I'll explain how.

Crystals have the ability to help us feel grounded and stable. Learn how to use crystals properly and you'll have less fear and anxiety in your life.

Crystals also work under the under the law of attraction, helping us to attract wealth and power into our lives.

I'll walk you through the steps of how to purchase crystals, cleanse and program them, and use them in your everyday life. Learn how to treat illnesses and attract love, success, and wealth with less fear in your life.

I welcome you on your journey to crystal healing.

How Do Crystals Heal

Energy is the essence of everything in the universe including the human body. In the same way, each crystal vibrates to a specific kind of energy. As you work with crystals, the crystal's energy blends with your own, transforming and amplifying the energy within your body. Sequentially, the crystals are also important as they assist in re-energizing and rebalancing your body on the emotional, spiritual, and physical levels.

Normally, each kind of crystal will radiate a particular type of energy that corresponds to and works with the specific energies in certain emotional and physical areas of yourself. Using crystals for healing is as simple as being around them. Other techniques may include holding a crystal in your hand or placing on a nightstand.

Since these healing crystals are constantly absorbing negative energy in order to provide healing, they can become blocked. Blockage will then reduce the healing effect of crystals; hence, making it important to cleanse. Cleansing releases the negative energy, which will recharge the stone and increase its healing power. In the following chapter, we will look at how you can cleanse and program your crystals.

Terminology In Crystal Healing

As you learn more about crystals and healing properties, you will come across various terms. We will look further into these terms in order to enable you to better understand crystal healing.

Programming

Crystals are said to have some kind of memory, owing to their repeating chemical structure. In other words, crystals can actually hold energies. Programming a crystal refers to putting a particular program to a crystal. You could be putting a program of love, protection or abundance, for instance, to the crystal. The crystal will then translate the kind of energy that you program it to release.

Cleansing

As explained earlier, crystals can hold memories. This ability enables them to remember negative as well as positive energy. Since crystals can hold energy, they need to be cleansed. If, for example, a crystal is placed in a room to get rid of negative energies like depression, this means that the crystal will take up some of the negative energies that it cleansed out of the room, hence the crystal will require cleansing. Cleansing refers to the "removal" of energies in a particular crystal.

Chunks

These are crystals that have notable facets. These stones are good for simply holding when meditating and even carrying in your pocket.

Clusters

These small crystals have been joined together naturally. Clusters are amazing for enriching a workplace or environment.

Tumblestones

Tumblestones are crystals that have been tumbled over each other several times with an increasingly finer abrasive until their sides become smooth and shiny.

Cut Crystals

As their name suggests, these are simply crystals that have been cut and polished into shapes, like spheres, wands, or pyramids, making the crystal very attractive. Actually, if crystals are well cut, the energy from the rock can be maintained and even in some cases amplified.

Single Terminated Wands

These crystals usually have a single point at one end and a rounded or rough edge on the other end. They are commonly used for healing and cleansing, as well as jewelry.

Healing Properties of Crystals

Crystals are known to possess different healing properties. In most cases, no singular crystal has only one purpose. Actually, a single stone will have multiple healing properties. We shall look at some of these healing properties and the different crystals that possess various healing properties.

Grounding Crystals

Each of one of us needs solid ground to stand on. Grounding crystals help the lofty person stay grounded and refrain from feeling lost in the world. A powerful grounding crystal will help root you and bring heightened awareness.

Shielding And Protective Crystals

Crystals can act as protective amulets or energy shields. Shielding and protective crystals are best when you wear or carry them. Since these crystals have great absorbing qualities, they need to be cleansed frequently to rid them of negative energies.

Chakra Balancing Crystals

All healing crystals usually have balancing energies. However, you need to determine where the imbalance is in order to know the specific type of stone to use in order to correct the balancing energies.

Love Crystals

These crystals carry warm and soft energies. These stones enable you to attract love and may help show you how to love yourself and become more compassionate with others.

Energizing Crystals

We may need to boost our energy from time to time. Energizing stones are a great way to get through tough times when you are feeling low. These crystals are powerful owing to their higher vibrations. These higher vibrations give off energy when you feel weak and fatigued. Since they are quite strong, they will need to be used sparingly. A great way of doing this is by wrapping them in a gold setting.

Meditation crystals

The use of crystals during meditating can help with focus. They are also helpful in assisting with the connection to a spiritual power source.

Manifesting Crystals

Manifesting stones are simply magical and can help you focus on the things you really want. They also enable you to maintain a positive mindset in order to manifest desires.

Record Keepers

Generally, all crystals are excellent at keeping memories. However, there are specific stones that are better at absorbing and retaining information. You can have these stones with you when attending a class, for instance. Rubies and garnets are known to help enable a person to remain grounded and focused during lectures. Carrying these stones in your pocket on examination days will help with your memory for the test.

How To Cleanse Crystals

Cleansing and programming of crystals is essential if you want to use the stones effectively for their healing properties.

Cleansing Crystals

Cleansing can be done daily, weekly, bi-weekly or monthly depending on how frequently you use the stone. Cleansing does not refer to the usual way of cleaning with water and soap; however, the goal of cleansing is to remove stored energies whether good or bad. Any crystals that will be used for healing need to be cleansed before and after use. Below are various cleansing methods that can be used.

Dry Salt

You may use dry salt without mixing it with water. Simply half-fill a glass bowl with sea salt or cooking salt and place the crystals into the salt. You can bury them in the salt or leave them on the surface for several hours or even days. You should then cleanse the crystals thoroughly with running cold water to remove any salt that may be remaining. Ensure that you throw away the salt and never reuse it, as it would have absorbed all of the negative energies.

Salt Water

You can leave crystals to soak in seawater or water that has been mixed with sea salt. If you are unable to get sea water/salt, you can also use cooking salt. Salt water cleansing is the best way to cleanse crystals. However, be aware that some crystals cannot be cleansed with salt water, as the salt water may change their appearance and even properties. Some common crystals that you can cleanse using seawater are those that contain metal, have water content, and are porous. Ensure that you do not use salt water to cleanse stones like Hematite, Pyrite, and Lapis Lazuli.

When cleansing, you should fill a glass bowl about ½ full with salt water then submerge the crystals in the water and leave them there for around 24 hours. If you need to do a deeper cleansing, you would need to leave them in the water for as long as a week.

Non-Contact Salt

This is one of the safest ways to cleanse crystals that may be damaged by salt. First fill a glass bowl with 2/3 dry sea salt. Put a smaller glass container into the glass with the salt. You can then place the crystals into the empty glass that is buried halfway in the dry salt. While this is a safe cleansing method, it will take longer as the salt does not have direct contact with the crystals and will have to draw the energies through the smaller glass.

Visualization

Thought energy, also known as visualization, is also effective in cleansing crystals. Hold the crystal and visualize a bright white light surrounding it, followed by a beam of white light that may be coming down through the stone and passing all the way through the crystal, ridding it of any stored energy. Do this until you are happy that the light has properly cleansed it.

Crystal Bed, Cluster, Geode or Druse

All crystals may be cleansed by placing them in a cluster, Geode, Druse or Bed. Place a few crystals onto the crystal points and leave them for up to 48 hours. These crystal cluster formations can absorb the energies contained in the crystal, neutralize them, and release good energy from the cluster into the crystals that you are cleansing.

Smudging

You may also use smudging to cleanse your crystals. This involves the burning of incense sticks or smudge sticks while holding the crystals in the smoke in order to cleanse the stored energies. The most suitable incense sticks are sweetgrass, sage, cedarwood, and sandalwood. Smudging of the crystals only takes about 30 seconds.

Programming Crystals

Once you get rid of energy from a crystal it will need it will need to be programed. It will especially need to be reprogrammed if you want it for a specific purpose beyond its general characteristics. When programming crystals for protection, activation of chakras or, healing, intention and focus are very important. Furthermore, when programming your crystals, you need to ensure that your stone is compatible with the specific purpose that you have in mind.

Meditation With Visualization

Meditation is quite common when it comes to programming crystals. When using this technique, sit in a quiet place, while holding the crystals in your hand, think about the specific purpose of the stone. As you move deeper into meditation, visualize how it would feel if your desire is fulfilled, focusing your programing and thought into the crystal. Repeat the program in your head several times until you feel that the crystal has absorbed your program. You will have to use and trust your intuition to know when the crystal has been programmed.

Meditation With Third-Eye Beaming

Using this method, you still follow the same instructions in the first method. Once you are in a meditative state, bring your cupped hands with the crystals up to your face at about eye level and imagine that you are beaming your program into the crystal using your third eye. Do this until you feel satisfied that the program is in the crystal.

Meditation With Breath

Follow the same instructions as the first method. Once you reach the meditative state, bring your cupped hands, with the crystals in them, up to your mouth then blow on your stone with your program in mind. This way, you are literally breathing your program into the crystal.

Meditation With Other Subtle Energy Techniques

Follow the same instructions as method one. Once you are in a meditative state, intend your program into the crystal. Repeat this until you feel the energy sensations in your hands have died down and you feel that the stone has been programmed sufficiently.

Usually, a crystal programmed for more active use will need to be programmed sooner, while one that has a more passive program can retain its program for a longer period of time. Therefore, crystals that are carried or worn need reprogramming much sooner than those left sitting in a particular place.

How To Purchase Crystals

While knowing the exact properties of a particular crystal may be helpful when shopping for these stones, it is not necessary for you to know all the properties. You should instead allow yourself to be drawn to a particular crystal. For instance, if you are at a shop in front of several crystals and are looking to buy one, just close your eyes, relax and when you open them, choose the one that you feel drawn to.

Shopping at a local store for crystals may allow you to touch the crystals, however, you may not be able to do that when looking for crystals online. You will need to rely on your intuition to choose a suitable crystal. You can browse at various pictures until you find the crystal that you feel drawn to. Some feel frustrated because of the inability to touch and feel the crystal and prefer to purchase them locally.

Your intent is usually important when purchasing items related to spiritual growth. As you buy crystals, its important to feel that a particular crystal strongly appeals to you and that you have an urge or feel drawn to that crystal. However, if you have no appeal to a particular crystal, you will have to accept that it is not the right time to buy the stone.

You may draw to buy a citrine crystal because it can dissipate negative energy, although you had intended on purchasing a different crystal. Follow your unconscious, since you will select the best crystal for a problem you did not realize that you have. Therefore, the best way of purchasing the most suitable crystal is to do what feels right.

Crystals For Attracting Wealth And Power

Did you know that you can attract wealth and power by simply using crystals? Various crystals have been known to be very effective in attracting wealth.

Citrine: This stone can attract abundance. You should put it at the furthest left corner of your house away from your front door. If by any chance this is the bathroom, do not put the stone there, as any wealth you get will go right down the toilet.

Green Aventurine, Jade and Emerald: You can wear or carry any of these stones. You may want to keep a green aventurine in your purse or wallet in order to multiply your money.

Malachite: This is a stone for not only abundance but also for purification, drawing out negative energies, and healing dreams. It also provides healing and positive transformation to the person wearing it.

Ruby: Ruby stimulates love that leads to nurturing, knowledge, health, spiritual wisdom, and wealth. Some people say that as long as you have a ruby, you will always be wealthy.

Pyrite: It is said that this stone is a symbol of good luck and money.

Peridot: This is simply known as stone money. Put a piece of it with citrine in your purse to increase your wealth.

Crystals To Reduce Fear And Anxiety

Do you get overly anxious when meeting new people or going to an interview? Using the crystals below can reduce or cause any anxiety or fear to dissipate.

Sunstone: This stone inspires independence, freedom, luck, and originality. It is also useful in dissipating fearfulness and alleviating stress. A sunstone will warm your heart and rejuvenate your spirit as it brings a sunny disposition.

Rose Quartz: This amazing crystal provides you emotional healing.

Aquamarine, Moonstone, Aventurine and Rhodonite: These stones are quite calming. You can lie down, place on your heart or massage yourself with them. You can even bath with them.

Black onyx, snowflake obsidian, chrysocolla, sodalite: You can use any of these stones to relieve fear, worry, anxiety and stress. Each time you feel that you are worried, you can take the stone, rub it between your fingers or wear it as jewelry. You may also massage with it.

Amber, Smoky quartz: When you feel depressed, any of these stones can be used.

Crystals For Other Ailments

In addition to attracting wealth and reducing fear and anxiety, crystals can be used to cure or provide relief for various ailments.

Headaches

The crystal that you will use to provide relief will depend on the cause of the headache. You can use amber, turquoise or amethyst for tension headaches. Lapis Lazuli is also quite effective for treating migraines.

Headaches may be caused due to an imbalance between head energy and solar plexus chakra, which may be brought on due to unsuitable food or stress. If this is the cause of your headache, you will need to look for a stone like moonstone and citrine that will balance your solar plexus chakra.

Difficulty Sleeping (Insomnia)

The kind of stone that you use to enable you to sleep will depend on the cause of the insomnia. If you think that the restlessness is due to overeating, you may need to use a stone like moonstone or iron pyrite to calm your stomach. If, however, you are having nightmares that are making it hard for you to sleep, you can place a stone line of tourmaline and smoky quartz at the foot of your bed.

In case tension and worry may be a hindrance to your sleep, you can place crystals like citrine, rose quartz and amethyst under your pillow to sooth and calm you.

Lack Of Libido

You can use red garnet or fluorite to stimulate passion and rid emotional conditions that may be blocking sexual energy.

Treating Pain

In case you have menstrual cramps, you can tape a carnelian to your lower abdomen to relieve the pain.

Bloodstone, malachite and Lapis are also amazing pain relievers. If you have any form of pain on any body part, you can place any of these stones to the specific area until the pain reduces.

Lack of Energy

If your energy levels are low, use yellow or orange crystals to increase your energy. Some of these crystals include golden amber, and deep red garnet.

Conclusion

Crystal healing is real and has worked for thousands of years. Rather than turning to medications, give crystal healing a try. Attract positive things into your life, improve insomnia, headaches, and more. I hope this book has started you on a healing crystal journey.

You May Enjoy My Other Books

Below you'll find some of my other popular books on Amazon. You can also visit my author page.

hyperurl.co/MarySolomon

HEARING GOD'S VOICE FOR BEGINNERS

smarturl.it/heargod

HEALING: Heal Your Body Heal Your Life

smarturl.it/healingaa

AFFIRMATIONS and ASCENDED MASTERS: Achieve A Higher Consciousness

hyperurl.co/affirmations

AUTOIMMUNE DISEASE ANTI-INFLAMMATORY DIET

smarturl.it/autoa

CHAKRA HEALING EXPOSED

smarturl.it/chakraaa

MEDICAL MARIJUANA and Pain Free Living

smarturl.it/mja

LAW OF ATTRACTION

smarturl.it/loaa

26247504R00056

Printed in Great Britain
by Amazon